Whole Body Reset Diet Cookbook
for Middle Aged

Tasty and Easy Recipes to Boost Your Metabolism, for a Flat Belly and Optimum Health at Midlife and Beyond

Marah Pattle

TABLE OF CONTENTS

INTRODUCTION

In 2012, Harley Pasternak, a celebrity fitness trainer who co-hosted ABC's daytime talk show "The Revolution," developed the Body Reset Diet. Pasternak has worked with many A-listers, including Ariana Grande, Alicia Keys, Lady Gaga, Gwyneth Paltrow, Adam Levine, Megan Fox, Rihanna, Kanye West, Bono, and Katy Perry.

The diet is divided into three phases, each lasting five days, and the first phase consists mostly of drinking smoothies before reintroducing solid foods. First, you'll only be consuming smoothies for your meals. That means you'll only be having smoothies as part of your meals throughout the first phase. Milk or Greek yoghurt is a wonderful source of protein, and white smoothies are a fantastic way to get it. For a quick rush of energy, try a red smoothie made with fruits, while a green smoothie made with veggies will keep you satisfied until dinnertime. A salad, sandwich or stir-fry can be substituted for one of your two smoothies each day during the second phase of the diet. Finally, in phase three, a substantial meal is substituted for one of the two smoothies.

It's a 15-day experiment to see if a low-calorie plant-based diet consisting mostly of smoothies may educate your body to burn calories more effectively while you sleep. With three days of resistance training a week, you'll be on your way to long-term weight loss.

There may be a greater food spending on the Body Reset Diet because you'll be eating many fruits and veggies. Since you won't be purchasing any meat or other solid foods for the first few weeks, you may experience a drop in your shopping price. Instead of buying fresh produce, Pasternak says, you can buy most fruits and vegetables pre-frozen and save money on groceries.

On the Body Reset Diet, you're likely to shed a few pounds. Unfortunately, dietary data does not exist for this diet; however, consuming only smoothies made from fresh produce may provide a deficit in calories, which might lead to weight loss. Whether or whether you manage to lose the weight and keep it off is entirely up to you.

Vegetarianism and the Body Reset diet both adhere to similar principles. As a general rule, vegetarians tend to consume fewer calories and weigh less than their meat-eating counterparts and eat a greater number of fruits and vegetables. Fruit and vegetable-rich diets have been linked to greater health in the long term.

BREAKFAST RECIPES

Green Goddess Smoothie

Preparation Time: 5 minutes

Cooking Time: 0 minutes

Servings: 1

Ingredients

- 1 ripe avocado, peeled and pitted
- 1 cup almond milk or water, plus more as needed
- 1 cup baby spinach leaves, stems removed
- ½ medium cucumber, peeled and seeded
- 1 tbsp olive oil or avocado oil
- 8 to 10 fresh mint leaves, stems removed
- Juice of 1 lime (about 1 to 2 tablespoons)

Directions

1. In a blender, combine the avocado, almond milk, spinach, cucumber, olive oil, mint, and lime juice.
2. Blend until smooth and creamy, adding more almond milk or water if necessary.

Breakfast Muffins

Preparation Time: 10 mins

Cooking Time: 30 mins

Servings: 8

Ingredients

- 4 eggs
- 4 slices bacon, chopped and cooked
- ½ cup of almond flour
- ½ cup salsa

Directions

1. Preheat oven to 350 ° degrees Fahrenheit. Cooking spray should be used to grease the muffin cups.

2. In a blender, mix eggs, bacon, almond flour, and salsa on medium speed for thirty seconds or until fully incorporated.

3. Fill muffin cups halfway with the mixture.

4. Bake for 30 minutes, or until a toothpick poked into the middle of a muffin comes out clean. Allow cooling for ten minutes before serving.

Blueberry Pancakes

This is a quick, tasty, high-protein breakfast that's also strong in antioxidants. It's highly customizable, and reducing the flour makes it paleo-friendly.

Preparation Time: 10 mins

Cooking Time: 10 mins

Servings: 2

Ingredients

- 1 ripe banana, cut into pieces
- 1 tbsp chia seeds
- 2 eggs
- ½ tsp dark cocoa powder (Optional)
- 1 tbsp all-purpose flour
- ½ tsp ground cinnamon (optional)
- 1 pinch of sea salt
- ½ tsp vanilla extract (optional)
- ¼ cup of blueberries
- 1 tbsp coconut oil or more as required

Directions

1. Add in chia seeds in a blender. Blend them until powdery for three to five seconds. Add eggs, banana, flour, cinnamon, cocoa powder, sea salt, and vanilla extract; blend, usually scraping sides down, till the batter is uniform and smooth.

2. Over medium heat, heat a skillet. Add coconut oil to the skillet. Pour half of the batter into the oil. Sprinkle half of the blueberries onto the batter. Then cook it until the bubbles are formed, and the edges are dried for about three to four minutes. Cook them while flipping until browned on both sides, for two to three minutes. Repeat with the leftover blueberries and batter by using coconut oil if required.

Green Tea Smoothie

Preparation Time: 5 minutes

Cooking Time: 0 minutes

Servings: 2

Ingredients

- 1 cup crushed ice, divided
- 1 cup unsweetened almond milk
- ¼ cup heavy (whipping) cream
- 1 tablespoon coconut oil
- 3 tablespoons unsweetened vanilla protein powder
- 1½ teaspoons green tea powder

Directions

1. Blend ½ cup of ice, almond milk, heavy cream, and coconut oil in a blender.
2. Add the vanilla protein powder, green tea powder, and the remaining ½ cup of ice. Blend for 1 minute, or until smooth, and serve.

High-Fiber Breakfast Bars

Preparation Time: 15 mins

Cooking Time: 30 mins

Servings: 12

Ingredients

- 1 ½ cups of oats
- Cooking spray
- ¼ cup of wheat germ
- 2 tbsp protein powder, vanilla-flavored hemp
- ¼ cup of ground flax seed
- 1 tsp ground cinnamon
- 3 bananas
- ½ tsp salt
- ¼ cup of peanut butter, or according to taste
- ¼ cup peanut butter
- 1 tsp vanilla extract
- 2 tbsp honey

Directions

1. Preheat the oven to 375°F. Spray an 8 by an 8-inch baking dish with cooking spray and line with aluminum foil, allowing foil to lie flat over the edges of the pan.

2. Combine wheat germ, oats, protein powder, flaxseed, salt, and cinnamon in a mixing bowl. In another mixing bowl, mash bananas and mix in 1/4 cup of peanut butter, vanilla extract, and honey until thoroughly combined. Mix the remaining ingredients (dry) into the banana mixture and lay it out in the baking dish that you've prepared.

3. Cook for twenty minutes in a preheated oven. On the top, spread 1/4 cup peanut butter.

4. Continue baking for another ten minutes till the center is firm and sides are gently browned. Allow cooling in the pan before lifting bars onto a cutting board using aluminum foil handles. Refrigerate after cutting into bars and wrapping with plastic wrap.

Protein Crepes

Preparation Time: 10 mins

Cooking Time: 10 mins

Servings: 2

Ingredients

- 1 cup skim milk
- 1 cup of whole wheat flour
- 1 pinch of ground cinnamon, or according to taste
- 4 egg whites
- 1 tsp ground cinnamon
- 1 tbsp olive oil
- Olive oil cooking spray
- 1 tbsp jelly
- 1 cup Greek yogurt, plain fat-free

Directions

1. In a big mixing bowl, mix milk, flour, olive oil, cinnamon, and egg whites until smooth.

2. Set a skillet over medium heat, lightly sprayed with cooking spray. Pour 1/4 cup batter onto the skillet and spin it, so the batter stretches out in a thin layer around the sides. Cook for approximately two minutes or until the bottom is gently browned. Cook for another two minutes on the other side, or until the bottom is gently browned. Continue with the remaining batter.

3. In a mixing dish, combine jelly and Greek yogurt. Fill each crepe with a layer of yogurt mixture and wrap it around the filling. Serve the remaining yogurt mixture on the plates' rolled crepes. Cinnamon should be sprinkled on each crepe.

Lemon High Protein Smoothie

Preparation Time: 5 minutes

Cooking Time: 0 minutes

Servings: 2

Ingredients

- 1 cup unsweetened almond milk
- ½ cup coconut milk
- 2 tablespoons egg white protein powder
- 1 teaspoon pure vanilla extract
- 1 teaspoon lemon extract
- 2 cups ice cubes

Directions

1. In a blender, blend the almond milk, coconut milk, egg white powder, vanilla, plus lemon extract, until combined.

2. Add the ice, blend until smooth and thick, and serve.

High-Protein Torte

Preparation Time: 20 mins

Cooking Time: 30 mins

Servings: 8

Ingredients

- Garbanzo beans, rinsed
- 1 (19 oz) can chickpeas
- 4 eggs
- 1 cup Splenda or sugar
- 1 (15 oz) can pumpkin
- 2 tbsp maple sugar
- 2 tsp pumpkin pie spice
- ¼ cup of walnut halves
- ½ tsp baking powder
- 6 oz whipped cream cheese
- 1 (11 oz) drained, can mandarin oranges
- 2 cups sugar, powdered

Directions

1. Preheat the oven to 350 °F. Mix eggs and chickpeas in a food processor or blender and mix until smooth. Blend again till smooth while adding the Splenda, pumpkin, syrup, spice, and baking powder.

2. Spray an 8-inch circular cake pan with cooking spray. Fill the cup halfway with batter. Bake for about sixty minutes, till a knife stabbed in the center comes out clean. Cool. Before taking out the cake from the pan, make sure it is entirely cool since it is extremely soft.

3. Combine the powdered sugar and cream cheese in a mixing bowl. Cover the sides and tops of the cake with the frosting. Walnuts and mandarin oranges may be used to decorate.

Quinoa Breakfast Bowl

Preparation Time: 5 mins

Cooking Time: 20 mins

Servings: 1

Ingredients

- ¼ cup quinoa, multi-colored
- ½ cup water
- ½ cup cottage cheese, reduced-sodium
- 1 tbsp fresh blueberries
- ½ sliced banana
- 1 pinch of ground cinnamon
- 1 tsp chia seeds

Directions

1. In a saucepan, boil the quinoa and water. Reduce the heat to medium-low. Cover and let them boil until the quinoa is tender for about fifteen to twenty minutes. Then let them cool.

2. Mix half cup cottage cheese and quinoa in a bowl. Add on banana, chia seeds, cinnamon, and blueberries. Mix them well and serve.

High-Protein Nutty Pasta

This may be a vegetarian, fast, nutritious, and tasty breakfast or supper when nothing else in the home would suffice. We're constantly looking for high-protein, quick-to-prepare meals, and this one is now the best. What's not to like about pasta? We usually have some on hand. Serve cold or hot with your favorite salad dressing and, if preferred, more sunflower seeds.

Preparation Time: 15 mins

Cooking Time: 20 mins

Servings: 4

Ingredients

- 1 (8 oz) package quinoa pasta
- 1 drizzle olive oil, extra-virgin
- ¼ cup tofu, diced
- 2 tbsp grated cheese blend, Parmesan-Romano
- 2 tbsp feta cheese, crumbled
- 2 tbsp chopped pecans
- 2 tbsp sunflower seeds, roasted
- 2 tbsp slivered or sliced almonds
- ½ teaspoon dried parsley
- 2 tbsp pimentos, minced
- Pepper and salt according to taste
- 1 tbsp butter

Directions

1. Bring a large saucepan of lightly salted water to a boil. Combine in olive oil and quinoa pasta. Boil for about thirteen to fifteen minutes, or until the pasta is cooked and firm to the bite. Drain the pasta and set it aside.

2. In a large salad bowl, combine feta cheese, tofu, Parmesan-Romano cheese, almonds, nuts, sunflower seeds, parsley, and pimentos. Mix the butter and hot pasta until the butter has melted.

Protein-Rich Peanut Butter Balls

This recipe creates 25 to 30 crunchy walnut-sized sweets that melt perfectly. Simply divide them among plastic zip lock bags and freeze them. You'll be prepared with a nutritious, high-protein snack rather than grabbing for a packaged box full of things you can't even spell.

Preparation Time: 20 mins

Cooking Time: 2 hrs

Servings: 25

Ingredients

- 2 scoops of protein powder, cocoa whey
- 2 cups peanut butter, crunchy
- 2 tbsp flax seeds
- 2 ripe and mashed bananas

Directions

1. Combine cocoa whey powder, peanut butter, flaxseed, and bananas in a big bowl.

2. In a walnut-size ball, squeeze in the mixture and put them in a tray covered with parchment (to separate the layers).

3. Freeze for about two hours before serving.

Protein-Rich Granola Bars

Preparation Time: 20 mins

Cooking Time: 12 mins

Servings: 12

Ingredients

- 1 cup canned chickpeas, drained
- cooking spray
- 2 egg whites
- 1 ½ cups rolled oats, old-fashioned
- 1 small and grated apple
- 1 cup wheat cereal, puffed
- ½ cup chocolate chips, mini semisweet
- ½ cup applesauce
- ¼ cup honey
- ¼ cup dried cranberries, sweetened
- ¼ cup of almond butter
- ½ teaspoon ground cinnamon
- ¼ cup chopped almonds

Directions

1. Preheat the oven to 350 degrees Fahrenheit.
2. Using cooking spray, grease a small muffin tray.
3. In a food processor, combine egg whites and chickpeas until thoroughly combined.
4. Fill a bowl halfway with the chickpea mixture. Stir in the oats, apple, puffed wheat, chocolate chips, applesauce, honey, cranberries, almond butter, cinnamon, and almonds until well combined.
5. Add the batter into prepared muffin tins and flatten with a fork.
6. Bake for about twelve minutes in a preheated oven until the edges are brown.

Strawberry Spinach Smoothie

Preparation Time: 5 minutes

Cooking Time: 0 minutes

Servings: 2

Ingredients

- 1 cup crushed ice, divided
- ½ cup unsweetened almond milk
- 2 cups fresh spinach
- ½ cup strawberries
- 1 tablespoon coconut oil

Directions

1. Blend ½ cup of ice, almond milk, spinach, strawberries, and coconut oil in a blender. Add the remaining ½ cup of ice.

2. Blend for 1 minute, or until smooth, and serve.

Avocado Blueberry Smoothie

Preparation Time: 5 minutes

Cooking Time: 0 minutes

Servings: 2

Ingredients

- 1 cup crushed ice, divided
- ½ cup blueberries
- ¾ cup unsweetened almond milk
- 2 tablespoons heavy (whipping) cream
- 1 tablespoon coconut oil
- 1 avocado, peeled and pitted

Directions

1. Blend ½ cup of ice, blueberries, almond milk, heavy cream, and coconut oil in a blender.

2. Add the avocado and remaining ½ cup of ice. Blend for 1 minute, or until smooth, and serve.

Eggs and Greens Dish

Preparation Time: 10 mins

Cooking Time: 10 mins

Servings: 2

Ingredients

- 1 tbsp olive oil
- 1 cup of fresh spinach
- 2 cups of chopped and stemmed rainbow chard
- ground black pepper and salt according to taste
- ½ cup of arugula
- 4 eggs, beaten
- 2 minced cloves of garlic
- ½ cup of shredded Cheddar cheese

Directions

1. Heat the oil in a skillet on a medium-high flame. Saute spinach, arugula, and chard till tender for 3 minutes. After that, add garlic; cook and stir till fragrant, for 2 minutes.

2. Mix cheese and eggs in a bowl, then pour into chard mixture. Coat and cook till set, for 5 to 7 minutes. Season with pepper and salt.

Triple Berry Smoothie

Preparation Time: 5 minutes

Cooking Time: 0 minutes

Servings: 2

Ingredients

- 1 cup crushed ice, divided
- ½ cup unsweetened almond milk
- 1 tablespoon coconut oil
- ½ cup blueberries
- ½ cup raspberries
- ½ cup blackberries
- ½ teaspoon pure vanilla extract

Directions

1. Blend the ½ cup ice, almond milk, and coconut oil in a blender.
2. Add the blueberries, raspberries, blackberries, vanilla, and remaining ½ cup of ice. Blend for 1 minute, or until smooth, and serve.

Eggs Florentine

Preparation Time: 10 mins

Cooking Time: 10 mins

Servings: 3

Ingredients

- 2 tbsp butter
- 2 minced cloves garlic
- 3 tbsp cream cheese, diced into small pieces
- ½ cup of mushrooms, diced
- ½ (10 oz.) package fresh spinach
- ground black pepper and salt according to taste
- 6 large eggs, beaten slightly

Directions

1. Melt the butter in a big skillet on a medium flame; cook and mix garlic and mushrooms till the garlic is fragrant, for about 1 minute. Then add spinach to the mushroom mixture and simmer till the spinach is wilted, for 2 to 3 minutes.

2. Stir the eggs into the mushroom-spinach mixture, then season with pepper and salt. Cook, without mixing, till the eggs begin to firm, flip. Sprinkle the cream cheese over the egg mixture and simmer till the cream cheese begins to soften for 5 minutes.

Caprese On Toast

Preparation Time: 15 mins

Cooking Time: 5 mins

Servings: 14

Ingredients

- 14 slices of sourdough bread
- 1 lb fresh mozzarella cheese, diced 1/4-inch thick
- 2 peeled cloves garlic
- ⅓ cup of fresh basil leaves
- 3 tbsp extra-virgin olive oil
- 3 large tomatoes, diced 1/4-inch thick
- ground black pepper and salt according to taste

Directions

1. Toast the bread slices, then rub each side of each slice with the garlic. Put a mozzarella cheese slice, a slice of tomato, and 1 to 2 basil leaves on each piece of toast. Then drizzle with olive oil and season with black pepper and salt.

Vegan Clam Chowder

Preparation Time: 5 minutes

Cooking Time: 40 minutes

Servings: 6-8

Ingredients

- 1 1/2 cups of Garbanzo Beans-cooked
- 1 1/2 cups of chopped Oyster Mushrooms*
- 2 cups of Garbanzo Bean Flour
- 1 cup of mashed White Onions
- 1/2 cup of chopped Butternut Squash
- 1/2 cup of medium diced Kale
- 1 cup of Homemade Hempseed Milk
- 1 cup of Aquafaba
- 2 teaspoons of Dill
- 1/2 teaspoon of Cayenne Powder
- 2 teaspoons of Basil
- 1 tablespoon of Pure Sea Salt
- 1 tablespoon of Grape Seed Oil
- 7 cups Water

Directions

1. Pour Aquafaba and 6 cups of Spring Water into a large pot.
2. Add cooked Garbanzo Beans, chopped vegetables, and half of each seasoning to the pot.
3. Bring to a rolling boil and cook on medium heat for 10 minutes, stirring occasionally.
4. Whisk Hempseed Milk, Grape Seed Oil, 1 cup of Spring Water and the rest of the seasonings in a separate bowl. Slowly whisk in the Chickpea Flour.
5. Continue adding the flour, whisking constantly, until it is fully combined and there are no lumps.
6. Slowly pour the mixture into the pot with vegetables and whisk to avoid lumps.
7. Add chopped Oyster Mushrooms and cook on low heat for 10 minutes. Stir the soup occasionally.
8. Serve and enjoy your Vegan Clam Chowder!

Basil Avocado Pasta

Preparation Time: 5 minutes

Cooking Time: 20 minutes

Servings: 4

Ingredients

- 4 cups of cooked Spelt pasta
- 1 medium diced Avocado
- 2 cups of halved Cherry Tomatoes
- 1 minced fresh Basil
- 1 teaspoon of Agave Syrup
- 1 tablespoon of Key Lime Juice
- 1/4 cup of Olive Oil

Directions

1. Place the cooked pasta in a huge bowl.
2. Add diced Avocado, halved Cherry Tomatoes, and minced Basil into the bowl.
3. Stir all the ingredients until well combined.
4. Whisk Agave Syrup, Olive Oil, Pure Sea Salt and Key Lime juice in a separate bowl. Pour it over the pasta and stir until well combined.

Lunch

Low-Carb Tacos

Preparation Time: 20 mins

Cooking Time: 15 mins

Servings: 4

Ingredients

- 1 onion, diced
- 1 half lbs ground beef
- ½ (4 oz) can jalapeno peppers, diced
- 2 cups lettuce, shredded
- 1 (1 oz) package taco (seasoning mix)
- 1 chopped tomato
- ¼ cup salsa
- ½ cup low-fat Cheddar cheese, shredded
- 1 avocado, pitted, sliced, and peeled
- ¼ cup sour cream, low-fat

Directions

1. In a pan over medium heat, cook and stir onion, ground beef, and jalapeño peppers till the beef mixture is crumbly and browned, for seven to ten minutes. Mix taco seasoning into the beef mixture, reduce to low heat, and cook for five minutes until flavors are blended.

2. Combine the shredded lettuce, beef mixture, tomato, salsa, sour cream, and Cheddar cheese in a large mixing bowl. Garnish each bowl with avocado slices and distribute taco mixture among them.

Breakfast Quinoa

Preparation Time: 10 mins

Cooking Time: 15 mins

Servings: 4

Ingredients

- ¼ cup of chopped raw almonds
- 1 cup of quinoa
- 1 tsp ground cinnamon
- 2 pitted, dried dates, chopped finely
- 2 cups of milk
- 1 tsp vanilla extract
- 1 tsp sea salt
- 2 tbsp honey
- 5 dried apricots, chopped finely

Directions

1. Toast almonds in a skillet on a medium flame till just golden, for 3 to 5 minutes; then put it aside.

2. In a saucepan, heat the quinoa and cinnamon together over medium flame until cooked through. Stir in the milk and salt in the saucepan; bring to a boil, reduce heat to a minimum, cover, and cook for 15 minutes at a low simmer. In a large mixing bowl, combine the honey, quinoa, dates, about half of the almonds, and apricots. To serve, sprinkle the remaining almonds on top.

Keto Salmon Curry

Salmon curry is a simple and tasty keto dish that anybody can prepare, even if they have no prior cooking expertise.

Preparation Time: 20 mins

Cooking Time: 15 mins

Servings: 2

Ingredients

- ½ medium, diced onion
- 2 tbsp coconut oil
- 2 cups green beans, diced
- 1 lb diced salmon fillets
- 2 cups of chicken stock
- 1 ½ tbsp curry powder
- 1 (14 oz) can of coconut milk, chilled and solid cream only
- 1 tsp garlic powder
- 2 tbsp fresh basil, chopped
- Ground black pepper and salt according to taste

Directions

1. Heat the coconut oil in a medium to high heat pot. Add the onions. Cook them until translucent for about five minutes. Mix in green beans and saute them for about three minutes until nearly tender. Add in stock and let it boil. Add curry powder, garlic powder, and salmon. Also mix in coconut cream, and reduce the heat. Let it simmer until the salmon flesh come off easily with a fork, for three to five minutes. Season with pepper and salt. Garnish with basil.

Whipped Cauliflower

Preparation Time: 10 mins

Cooking Time: 10 mins

Servings: 4

Ingredients

- ¼ cup of Parmesan cheese
- 1 head cauliflower, dice into florets
- 1 tbsp cream cheese
- 2 tsp roasted garlic, or according to taste
- 2 tsp chicken soup base
- 1 ½ tsp butter
- Ground black pepper and salt according to taste
- ½ tsp milk, or according to taste (Optional)

Directions

1. Boil a pot of water. Cook the cauliflower florets in boiling water for about ten minutes. Cook them until they are tender; then drain in a strainer. Place some paper towels on the cauliflower's top and gently press down with the back of a big bowl to extract as much juice as possible.

2. Combine cream cheese, Parmesan cheese, chicken soup base, butter, and roasted garlic in a mixing bowl. In the cheese mixture, add the cauliflower and beat with a mixer for about three minutes, or until it is creamy. Mix in the milk until you get the desired texture. Add pepper and salt according to taste.

Bum's Lunch

Preparation Time: 15 mins

Cooking Time: 45 mins

Servings: 4

Ingredients

- 4 potatoes, medium and thinly sliced
- 4 (4 oz) cube steaks
- 1 large, thinly sliced onion
- Salt and pepper according to taste
- 4 tsp margarine

Directions

1. Preheat the oven to 350°F

2. 4 squares of aluminum foil must be set down. Place 1 cube steak on each foil sheet. Season the steaks with pepper and salt after spreading margarine over them. Over each steak, place one sliced potato and a couple of onion rings. If desired, season with pepper and salt once more. Wrap the foil of all-around food and seal it to make a packet. Packets should be placed on a baking pan.

3. In a preheated oven, bake for forty-five minutes, just until the beef is no pinker and the potatoes are soft. Open with caution since hot steam will be emitted.

High-Temp Pork Roast

Preparation Time: 15 mins

Cooking Time: 1 hr

Servings: 8

Ingredients

- ¼ cup of Worcestershire sauce
- 2 lbs pork roast
- 2 tsp ground black pepper, coarse
- 1 tsp Montreal steak seasoning
- 1 tsp sea salt, coarse
- ½ tsp garlic powder
- 1 tsp onion powder

Directions

1. Preheat oven to 500 degrees Fahrenheit.

2. To wet the outside of the roast, rinse it under cold running water. Allow to air dry. Spread Worcestershire sauce uniformly over the outside using a brush or paper towel. On both sides, season the roast with salt, pepper, steak seasoning, garlic powder, and onion powder.

3. Place the roast fat-side up in a wide roasting pan on the center rack.

4. Roast for twenty minutes for medium, twenty-four minutes for medium-well, and twenty-eight minutes for well done in a preheated oven until done to your liking. Switch off the oven and let the roast in for another forty minutes without opening the door.

5. Remove the pan from the oven and wrap it loosely with foil. Enable a 10- to 15-minute rest period to allow the liquids to settle back into the roast. Serve thinly sliced.

Chicken & Bacon Caesar Salad

Preparation Time: 10 mins

Cooking Time: 25 mins

Servings: 6

Ingredients

- 4 tablespoons olive oil
- 4 chicken breasts, skin on or off
- ½ ciabatta loaf, cubed
- 1 large cos (or Romaine) lettuce, leaves separated
- 75 g (3 oz) cooked crispy bacon rashers, broken into pieces
- 6 tablespoons Caesar salad dressing
- 25 g (1 oz) Parmesan cheese shavings
- Salt and pepper

Directions

1. The water oven must be filled and preheated to 65 °C (149 °F).

2. In a big, heavy-based frying pan, heat 2 tablespoons of oil. Season the chicken breasts with salt and pepper and sear over medium-high heat for 1–2 minutes on each side until golden. Remove from the pan, cool slightly, then divide a single layer between 2 small cooking pouches. Vacuum seal at the sealer's natural/dry setting and submerge for 1 hour.

3. Meanwhile, put the ciabatta cubes on a foil-lined grill pan and drizzle over the remaining olive oil. Toast for about 5 minutes under a preheated medium grill, turning periodically until golden and crisp.

4. Withdraw and set aside. Remove from their pouches the chicken breasts, pat dry with kitchen paper, and slice into bite-sized bits.

5. Tear the lettuce leaves roughly and put them with the chicken and most bacon bits in a salad bowl. Apply the salad dressing and toasted bread cubes and toss well to match. Sprinkle and serve immediately over the reserved bacon bits and the Parmesan shavings.

Barbecued Poussins with Chili Corn Salsa

Preparation Time: 10 mins

Cooking Time: 45 mins

Servings: 4

Ingredients

- finely grated rind and juice of 1 lime
- 2 tbsp Cajun spice mix
- 3 tbsp olive oil
- 2 poussins, each jointed in half and flattened slightly, 5 cm (2 inches) thick
- 175 g (6 oz) can sweetcorn
- 1 red chili, finely chopped
- ¼ cucumber, finely chopped
- Salt and pepper

Directions

1. The water oven must be filled and preheated to 65 °C (149 °F).

2. The turkey fillets are seasoned with salt and pepper and divided into 2 small cooking pouches. Vacuum seal at the sealer's natural/dry environment and submerge for 11/2 hours.

3. Meanwhile, heat the oil in a big, heavy-based frying pan over medium heat and cook the garlic for a few seconds. Passata, sugar, and oregano are added. Simmer until thick and pulpy for 5-8 minutes, then, if the frying pan is not ovenproof, pour into a small, ovenproof gratin dish. Take the turkey fillets out of their pouches and place them on the tomato sauce.

4. Mix half of the Parmesan with the breadcrumbs, then scatter over the turkey fillets. Once the cheese has melted, and the sauce is bubbling, scatter over the mozzarella and remaining Parmesan and position under a preheated grill for 2-3 minutes. If needed, serve with crusty bread.

Scrumptious Chicken

Preparation Time: 10 mins

Cooking Time: 25 mins

Servings: 6

Ingredients

- 2 tsp olive oil
- 2 tbsp white wine
- 6 skinless, chicken breast boneless halves
- 3 minced cloves garlic
- ½ cup of diced onion
- 3 cups of chopped tomatoes
- ½ cup of white wine
- 2 tsp fresh thyme chopped
- 1 tbsp fresh basil chopped
- ½ cup of kalamata olives
- ¼ cup of fresh parsley chopped
- salt & pepper for taste

Directions

1. In a wide skillet on medium heat, heat some oil & white wine. Sauté chicken for roughly 4-6 minutes on either side or till it's golden. Chicken should be extracted out of the skillet and put aside.

2. Sauté garlic for almost 30 seconds in the pan drippings and add onion & sauté for almost 3 minutes. Take to a simmer & add tomatoes. Reduce to a low flame, add white wine, & cook for almost 10 mins. Continue simmering for almost 5 mins longer with the thyme & basil.

3. Cover & return chicken to the skillet. Reduce to low heat & continue cooking till your chicken is completely cooked & no more pink color inside. Cook for around 1 min with the olives & parsley in the skillet. Season to taste with salt & pepper and serve.

Mediterranean Frittata

Preparation Time: 15 mins

Cooking Time: 40 mins

Servings: 4

Ingredients

- 3 tomato halves sun-dried
- 2 tsp olive oil extra-virgin
- ¼ yellow minced onion
- 5 cloves minced garlic
- ½ cup of chopped spinach frozen
- 1 (4.5 oz) can of drained sliced mushrooms
- 3 oz crumbled feta cheese
- 6 whites of egg
- ¼ cup of skim milk
- ¼ tsp salt
- ¼ tsp black pepper ground
- ¼ tsp dried basil
- 2 tbsp Parmesan cheese shredded

Directions

1. Preheat your oven to 350°F. Grease an 8" circular cake pan with cooking oil.
2. Rehydrate sun-dried tomatoes in a bowl full of warm water for around 10 minutes. Wash & finely cut.
3. In the medium skillet on medium flame, heat some olive oil; cook and mix onion & garlic until translucent, around 10 mins. Cook & mix spinach until it has thawed & the water has evaporated around 5 mins. In a large mixing bowl, combine sun-dried tomatoes, mushrooms, & feta cheese until well combined.
4. Whisk together salt, pepper, skim milk, egg whites, & basil until frothy. Stir spinach mix and Parmesan cheese in the egg mix carefully. Fill the ready pan halfway with the mixture sprinkle with the rest of the Parmesan cheese.
5. Bake in your oven for approximately 25 mins, or until the frittata appears set & browned over the top.

Mediterranean Wrap

Preparation Time: 25 mins

Cooking Time: 10 mins

Servings: 4

Ingredients

- 1 sliced red onion
- 1 sliced zucchini
- 1 sliced eggplant
- ¼ lb. sliced fresh mushrooms
- 1 sliced red pepper
- 1 tbsp olive oil
- salt & black pepper for taste
- 4 tortillas whole grain
- ¼ cup of goat cheese
- ¼ cup of basil pesto
- 1, sliced large avocado

Directions

1. In a wide container with a tight-fitting lid, combine the eggplant, mushrooms, onion, zucchini, & bell pepper. Season with pepper and salt. Drizzle some olive oil on the vegetables. Shake it to coat after closing the lid.

2. Over medium flame, heat the skillet or grill pan. Put your seasoned vegetables in skillet, mix, then cook for approximately 10 mins, or until tender.

3. Spread goat cheese & pesto on each tortilla. Divide the avocado slices evenly between the tortillas & cover with the vegetables. Each tortilla's bottom half should be folded and wrapped into a tight wrap.

Branzino Mediterranean

Preparation Time: 15 mins

Cooking Time: 25 mins

Servings: 4

Ingredients

- 2 tbsp divided olive oil
- 1 chopped red onion
- salt & black pepper for taste
- 3 whole Branzino fish, cleaned
- 2 wedges of fresh lemon
- 2 sprigs of fresh rosemary
- ½ cup of white wine
- ¼ cup of lemon juice
- 1 tbsp oregano leaves fresh
- ¼ cup of Italian parsley chopped
- 3 lemon wedges

Directions

1. Preheat your oven to around 325°F (165°C).
2. In a big baking pan, drizzle 1 tbsp olive oil; add onion & season with pepper and salt.
3. Stuff, all cavities of the two, washed fish with one lemon wedge, one rosemary sprig, & some red onions. Over both fish, drizzle white wine & lemon juice, then sprinkle with some oregano. Drizzle 1 tbsp olive oil on both fish.
4. Bake for around 25 mins, or until the fish becomes opaque, then quickly flakes using a fork. Separate fish by gently sliding a spatula through the bones; detach all bones. Arrange fish over the platter and sprinkle parsley & lemon wedges on top.

Black Olive Bread

Preparation Time: 30 mins

Cooking Time: 30 mins

Servings: 15

Ingredients

- 3 cups of bread flour
- 2 tsp dry yeast active
- 2 tbsp white sugar
- 1 tsp of salt
- ½ cup of black olives chopped
- 3 tbsp olive oil
- 1 ¼ cups of warm water
- 1 tbsp cornmeal

Directions

1. Combine flour, yeast, olive oil, sugar, black olives, salt, & water in a big mixing bowl.

2. Turn dough out onto the floured table. Knead for 5-10 mins, until it's smooth & elastic. Set aside and allow to double in size for approximately 45 minutes. Take a blow. Knead vigorously once more for about 5-10 minutes. Leave roughly 30 mins for the dough to double in size.

3. On the kneading surface, shape the dough into a circle. Invert the bowl and line with the lint-free and well-floured towel. Allow doubling in width.

4. When your bread is growing for the 3rd time, prepare the oven by placing a pan full of water into the bottom. Preheat your oven to 500°F.

5. Gently transform loaf out over a finely oiled and cornmeal-dusted sheet tray.

6. Bake loaf for around 15 mins at 500° F. Reduce oven temperature to 375° F. Bake for the next 30 mins, or till finished.

Dinner

Vegetarian Fried Rice

Preparation Time: 15 mins

Cooking Time: 10 mins

Servings: 6

Ingredients

- ½ (12 oz) package cubed firm tofu
- 1 tbsp olive oil
- 2 carrots, diced and peeled
- ¼ minced onion
- 2 diced stalks of celery
- 2 minced cloves garlic
- 3 cups white rice, cooked
- Black pepper and salt according to taste
- 1 (8 oz) package spinach, frozen, chopped and thawed
- 4 beaten eggs
- 1 tsp sriracha hot sauce

Directions

1. Heat the oil in a pan over medium heat. Add carrots, tofu, celery, garlic, and onion; stir and cook until vegetables are tender; for five to ten minutes. Season with pepper and salt.

2. Stir rice, spinach, and egg into the tofu mixture till the egg is no more runny, for about five minutes. Add in sriracha, season pepper, and salt.

Vegetable Sheet Pan and Shrimp Dinner

Preparation Time: 15 mins

Cooking Time: 20 mins

Servings: 4

Ingredients

- 1 red, chopped bell pepper
- One red, coarsely chopped onion
- 1 cup of diced fresh mushrooms
- 3 tbsp olive oil, divided
- 1 zucchini, chopped
- freshly ground black pepper and salt to taste
- 1 lb fresh shrimp, deveined and peeled
- ¼ tsp paprika
- ½ tsp garlic powder
- 1 tsp lemon zest

Directions

1. Preheat oven to 425 degrees F.
2. Combine bell pepper, red onion, mushrooms, 2 tbsp olive oil, zucchini, salt, paprika, and pepper on a sheet pan and mix well.
3. Roast in a preheated oven till the vegetables are softened for about fifteen minutes.
4. Meanwhile, the vegetables are roasting, mix 1 tbsp olive oil, shrimp, lemon zest, salt, pepper, and garlic powder in a bowl. Toss to mix well.
5. Take off the roasted vegetables from the oven and combine shrimp into the sheet pan, distributing everything out uniformly in one layer. Move back to the oven and bake till the shrimp are cooked through and are pink for five to seven minutes.

Soft Dinner Rolls

Preparation Time: 10 mins

Cooking Time: 15 mins

Servings: 15

Ingredients

- 1 cup warm water
- 3 ¼ cups of bread flour
- ¼ cup white sugar
- 2 tbsp melted butter
- 2 tbsp butter, softened
- 1 egg, large
- 1 tsp salt
- 1 tbsp active dry yeast

Directions

1. Using butter, grease a 9 by 13-inch baking dish.

2. In the pan of your bread machine, combine water, bread flour, sugar, egg, 2 tbsp softened butter, salt, and yeast in the sequence indicated by the manufacturer. Press 'Start' after selecting the Dough cycle. Remove the dough once the cycle is finished and push down to deflate it.

3. Form the dough into fifteen equal pieces and roll them out. Place rolls in a prepared baking dish, garnish with melted butter, and loosely cover with plastic wrap; let rise for thirty minutes or until doubled in volume.

4. Preheat your oven to 375 degrees Fahrenheit.

5. Bake rolls till golden brown on top for twelve to fifteen minutes in a preheated oven.

Easy Dinner Hash

Preparation Time: 15 mins

Cooking Time: 20 mins

Servings: 2

Ingredients

- 8 oz Italian sausage, bulk
- 1 tbsp vegetable oil
- 1 potato, diced and peeled
- 1 cup mixed vegetables, frozen
- ¼ chopped onion
- ¼ cup Cheddar cheese, shredded
- Pepper and salt according to taste

Directions

1. In a big skillet, heat the vegetable oil over low-medium heat. Add in the sausage. Cook until just slightly pink and crumbly, for about five minutes. Mix in the onion and diced potato. Continue to cook till the potatoes are lightly browned and soft, for ten to fifteen minutes.

2. Once they are cooked, mix in vegetables until hot. Add pepper and salt according to taste. Garnish with Cheddar cheese and serve.

Spice-Rubbed Ribs

Preparation Time: 10 mins

Cooking Time: 1 hour

Servings: 10

Ingredients

- 3 tbsp paprika
- 2 tbsp plus 1 tsp salt
- 2 tbsps plus 1 tsp garlic powder
- 2 tbsp cayenne pepper
- 4 tsp onion powder
- 4 tsp dried oregano
- 4 tsp dried thyme
- 4 tsp pepper
- 10 pounds pork baby back ribs

Instructions

1. Combine the ingredients in a small dish; rub over the ribs.

2. Utilize a drip pan to prepare the grill for indirect cooking. Covered, grill ribs for 1 hour or until meat is cooked, flipping periodically.

Popcorn Shrimp

Preparation Time: 20 mins

Cooking Time: 15 minutes

Servings: 6

Ingredients

- 1 pound small shrimp peeled and deveined
- 1 1/4 cups of all-purpose flour
- 2 tsp salt plus more for serving
- 1/2 tsp paprika smoked or regular
- 1/4 tsp pepper
- 1/4 tsp garlic powder
- 1 egg
- 1/4 cup of milk
- vegetable oil for frying
- 2 tsp chopped fresh parsley

Instructions

1. Combine the flour, salt, paprika, pepper, and garlic powder in a medium bowl.
2. To start, pat the shrimp dry and put them in a big bowl. Toss in 1/4 cup of the flour mixture until all shrimp are coated.
3. In a big deep pot, heat 3-4 inches of oil to 375 degrees F.
4. Whisk together the egg and milk in a small bowl.
5. Each shrimp should be dipped into the milk mixture and dusted with the remaining seasoned flour.
6. 8-10 shrimp chunks in the oil Cook, occasionally stirring, for 2-3 minutes, or until golden brown.
7. To drain the shrimp, take them out of the oil and put them on a paper towel. Rep with the remaining shrimp.
8. Serve immediately with chopped parsley.

Easy Shrimp Dinner

Preparation Time: 20 mins

Cooking Time: 15 mins

Servings: 8

Ingredients

- 3 cubes of chicken bouillon
- 2 ½ cups water
- 3 lbs shrimp, deveined and peeled
- ¼ cup soy sauce
- ⅓ cup green onion, chopped
- Salt according to taste
- ¼ cup cold water
- ¼ cup cornstarch
- 4 small tomatoes, diced and ripped
- 12 oz snow peas, trimmed

Directions

1. In a big saucepan, boil the water over medium heat. Add bouillon in boiling water. Mix in green onion, shrimp, salt, and soy sauce. Boil for three minutes.

2. Dissolve the cornstarch in cold water. Stir into the mixture of shrimp. Let it cook till the gets thick, then add snow peas and tomatoes. Serve.

Savory Oatmeal with Mushrooms

Preparation Time: 15 mins

Cooking Time: 4 hours 10 minutes

Servings: 4

Ingredients

- 1 cup steel-cut oats
- 8 ounces brown mushrooms, sliced
- 1/2 medium onion, chopped
- 1/2 teaspoon ground black pepper
- 1/2 teaspoon cayenne pepper
- 4 cups water
- 1/2 teaspoon sea salt
- 2 tablespoons grapeseed oil
- 4 cloves garlic, minced
- 3 sprigs fresh thyme
- 1 cup baby spinach

Directions

1. To 175 degrees F, preheat the sous vide water bath.
2. Place cooking pouches with steel-cut oats, water, salt, black pepper, and cayenne pepper; seal firmly.
3. In the water bath, submerge the cooking pouches; boil for 4 hours; reserve.
4. In a pan that is preheated over a medium-high flame, heat the oil. Sauté, until softened, the mushrooms, onion, and garlic.
5. Now, add some new thyme and proceed to cook for another 5 minutes. Spoon a blend of mushrooms over the cooked oatmeal. Top with spinach for babies and serve wet. Bon appétit!

Lemon Rosemary Salmon

Preparation Time: 10 mins

Cooking Time: 20 minutes

Servings: 2

Ingredients

- 1 lemon, thinly sliced
- 4 sprigs of fresh rosemary
- 2 salmon fillets, bones, and skin removed
- coarse salt as need
- 1 tbsp olive oil, or as needed

Instructions

1. 400°F oven (200 degrees C).

2. In a baking dish, arrange half of the lemon slices in a single layer. Top with 2 rosemary sprigs and salmon fillets—Season salmon with salt and top with remaining rosemary sprigs and lemon wedges. Drizzle with extra virgin olive oil.

3. Bake for twenty minutes, or until the fish is readily flaked with a fork.

SMALL MEALS

Ground Beef Hash

Preparation Time: 15 minutes

Cooking Time: 15-20 minutes

Servings: 6

Ingredients

- 4 tablespoons avocado oil
- 2 cups roughly chopped cauliflower
- 1/4 cup chopped yellow onion
- 1 tablespoon minced jalapeño
- 1 1/2 pounds ground beef
- 1 teaspoon granulated garlic
- 1 teaspoon granulated onion
- 1 teaspoon salt
- 1 teaspoon freshly ground black pepper
- 1/2 teaspoon dried parsley

Directions

1. Heat avocado oil in your medium skillet over high heat. Allow the oil to get hot, then add cauliflower.

2. Stir once to coat, then let cauliflower sit undisturbed for 2 minutes, watching closely to ensure it doesn't burn. Stir again, and then let cauliflower sit 2 more minutes.

3. Adjust the heat down to medium and add onions and jalapeños. Cook until softened, about 4 minutes.

4. Add beef, spices, and herbs and cook until meat is no longer pink about 7 minutes. Remove from heat and serve!

Loaded Barbecue Roasted Cabbage Steaks

Preparation Time: 10 minutes

Cooking Time: 35 minutes

Servings: 2

Ingredients

- ½ head cabbage, sliced into 4 (1-inch-thick) steaks
- 2 tablespoons avocado oil
- 1 teaspoon freshly ground black pepper
- ½ teaspoon sea salt
- 2 tablespoons sugar-free barbecue sauce
- 1 avocado, diced
- ½ jalapeño, seeded and thinly sliced
- 1 scallion, chopped
- 2 tablespoons sour cream
- ½ cup chopped fresh cilantro

Directions

1. Warm the oven to 400 F. Line a baking sheet with parchment paper.
2. Drizzle both sides of the cabbage steaks with the oil and season with pepper and salt.
3. Bake for 15 minutes, then flip and bake for 15 minutes. The cabbage should be browned with a tender center. Remove the cabbage steaks and turn the oven to broil.
4. Dividing evenly, top each cabbage steak with the barbecue sauce. Broil for 3 to 5 minutes.
5. Plate 2 steaks per serving and top with the avocado, jalapeño, scallion, sour cream, and cilantro.

Steak Bites and Zucchini Noodles

Preparation Time: 15 minutes

Cooking Time: 15 minutes

Servings: 4

Ingredients

- 3 tbsp olive oil
- 4 garlic cloves, peeled and minced
- 1 tbsp soy sauce
- ½ tsp garlic powder
- ½ tsp paprika
- ½ tsp black pepper
- 18 oz sirloin steak, diced
- 3 zucchinis, spiralized

Directions

1. Heat 2 tbsp olive oil in your frying pan and add the garlic. Cook for 5 minutes until fragrant.

2. Stir in the soy sauce, garlic powder, paprika, and black pepper. Set aside to cool while you prepare the rest of the dish.

3. Heat the remaining 1 tbsp olive oil in the pan and add the diced steak. Cook for 3/4 minutes on each side until the steak is almost cooked.

4. Pour the sauce into the pan and continue cooking for 1 further minute, stirring to coat the steak in the sauce fully.

5. If desired, heat the zucchini noodles or serve them cold alongside the steak bites.

Grilled Beef Burger on a Mushroom Bun

Preparation Time: 15 minutes

Cooking Time: 10 minutes

Servings: 4

Ingredients

- 14 oz minced beef
- 1 tsp paprika
- 2 tbsp BBQ sauce
- 2 tbsp olive oil
- 4 large mushrooms
- 1 onion, sliced
- 4 cherry tomatoes, sliced
- Handful lettuce
- 1 avocado, peeled and sliced

Directions

1. Mix the minced beef, paprika, and BBQ sauce in a bowl. Form into 4 even patties.
2. Heat 1 tbsp olive oil in your large skillet and cook the mushrooms for 5 minutes on either side until slightly browned and crispy.
3. Remove the mushrooms from the pan and heat the remaining 1 tbsp olive oil in the pan.
4. Add the beef burgers and onion. Cook within 4-5 minutes on either side until the beef has browned and the onions are translucent.
5. Create your burgers by placing the mushrooms on a plate and topping each with a beef burger, cherry tomatoes, lettuce, and avocado slices.
6. Add some more BBQ sauce and paprika for extra flavor. Serve and enjoy!

Jambalaya Squash Ribbons

Preparation Time: 25 minutes

Cooking Time: 20 minutes

Servings: 4

Ingredients

- 2 tablespoons unsalted butter
- 1 small yellow onion, sliced into half-moons
- 2 medium yellow squash, thinly sliced
- 2 medium zucchinis, thinly sliced
- 1 medium carrot, peeled and julienned
- 1 medium red bell pepper, seeded & julienned
- 1 medium green bell pepper, seeded & julienned
- 1 medium tomato, diced
- 1 cup raw edamame, shelled
- 1 tablespoon minced garlic
- 1 tablespoon Cajun seasoning
- ½ cup dry white wine
- 3 cups vegetable stock
- ¼ cup chopped fresh flat-leaf parsley

Directions

1. Heat your large skillet over high heat until it starts to give off a little smoke.
2. Add the butter and let it dissolved, then add the onion, yellow squash, zucchini, carrot, red and green bell peppers, tomato, edamame, garlic, and Cajun seasoning.
3. Cook, stirring often, until the vegetables pick up some color, about 6 minutes.
4. Deglaze your pan using the wine and add the stock. Add the parsley and cook until the liquid is reduced by half, about 10 minutes. Serve warm.

Spinach Pie

Preparation Time: 15 minutes

Cooking Time: 30 minutes

Servings: 6

Ingredients

- 2 tablespoons olive oil
- 1 medium yellow onion, peeled and chopped
- 1 (16-oz) package frozen spinach, chopped, thawed & drained
- 1/4 cup chopped scallions
- 1/8 teaspoon ground nutmeg
- 1 teaspoon garlic salt
- 6 large eggs, beaten

Directions

1. Warm the oven to 350 F. Lightly grease a 9" pie plate.
2. Heat olive oil in a skillet over medium heat. Add onion and cook until softened, within 4 minutes. Add spinach and cook until heated through, within 3 more minutes.
3. Combine the remaining ingredients in a medium bowl. Add spinach mixture and stir to mix well.
4. Pour the prepared mixture into a pie plate and bake for 30 minutes or until eggs have set.

Curry and Grape Chicken Salad Lettuce Cups

Preparation Time: 15 minutes

Cooking Time: 15 minutes

Servings: 2

Ingredients

- 1 (6- to 8-ounce) boneless, skinless chicken breast, cut into ¼-inch cubes
- ¼ cup mayonnaise
- 2 tablespoons sour cream
- 2 tablespoons halved red grapes
- 1 tablespoon sliced almonds, toasted
- 1 teaspoon curry powder
- ¼ teaspoon sea salt
- 1/8 teaspoon ground white pepper
- 6 butter lettuce leaves

Directions

1. In a medium skillet or saucepan, combine the chicken and enough water to come halfway up the chicken.

2. Let it low simmer over medium-high heat, cover, and cook the chicken for 10 to 15 minutes until the juices run clear.

3. Drain the poaching liquid and place the chicken in the refrigerator to cool for 15 to 20 minutes.

4. Mix the cooled chicken, mayonnaise, sour cream, grapes, almonds, curry powder, salt, and white pepper in a medium bowl until well incorporated.

5. Set 3 lettuce leaves each on two plates. Evenly divide the chicken salad among the lettuce leaves, taco-style, and serve.

Veggie Bowls

Preparation Time: 10 minutes

Cooking Time: 5 minutes

Servings: 4

Ingredients

- 1 tablespoon olive oil
- 1-pound asparagus, trimmed and roughly chopped
- 3 cups kale, shredded
- 3 cups Brussels sprouts, shredded
- ½ cup hummus
- 1 avocado, peeled, pitted, and sliced
- 4 eggs, soft boiled, peeled, and sliced

For the dressing:

- 2 tablespoons lemon juice
- 1 garlic clove, minced
- 2 teaspoons Dijon mustard
- 2 tablespoons olive oil
- Salt and black pepper to the taste

Directions

1. Heat your pan with 2 tablespoons of oil over medium-high heat, add the asparagus and sauté for 5 minutes, stirring often.

2. Combine the other 2 tablespoons of oil in a bowl with the lemon juice, garlic, mustard, salt, and pepper, and whisk well.

3. In a salad bowl, combine the asparagus with the kale, sprouts, hummus, avocado, and eggs and toss gently. Add the dressing, toss and serve.

SOUPS AND SALADS

Spinach and Kale Soup

Preparation Time: 5 minutes

Cooking Time: 5 minutes

Servings: 2

Ingredients

- 3 ounces vegan butter
- 1 cup fresh spinach, chopped coarsely
- 1 cup fresh kale, chopped coarsely
- 1 large avocado
- 3 tablespoons chopped fresh mint leaves
- 3½ cups coconut cream
- 1 cup vegetable broth
- Salt and black pepper to taste
- 1 lime, juiced

Directions

1. Melt the vegan butter in your medium pot over medium heat and sauté the kale and spinach until wilted, 3 minutes. Turn the heat off.

2. Stir in the remaining ingredients, and using an immersion blender, puree the soup until smooth. Dish the soup and serve warm.

Tofu and Mushroom Soup

Preparation Time: 15 minutes

Cooking Time: 10 minutes

Servings: 4

Ingredients

- 2 tablespoons olive oil
- 1 garlic clove, minced
- 1 large yellow onion, finely chopped
- 1 teaspoon freshly grated ginger
- 1 cup vegetable stock
- 2 small potatoes, peeled and chopped
- ¼ teaspoon salt
- ¼ teaspoon black pepper
- 2 (14-oz.) silken tofu, drained and rinsed
- 2/3 cup baby Bella mushrooms, sliced
- 1 tablespoon chopped fresh oregano
- 2 tablespoons chopped fresh parsley to garnish

Directions

1. Heat the olive oil in your medium pot over medium heat and sauté the garlic, onion, and ginger until soft and fragrant.

2. Pour in the vegetable stock, potatoes, salt, and black pepper. Cook until the potatoes soften, 12 minutes.

3. Stir in the tofu and using an immersion blender, puree the ingredients until smooth.

4. Mix in the mushrooms and simmer with the pot covered until the mushrooms warm up while occasionally stirring to ensure that the tofu doesn't curdle, 7 minutes.

5. Stir oregano, and dish the soup. Garnish with the parsley and serve warm.

Chilled Avocado Soup

Preparation Time: 50 minutes

Cooking Time: 0 minutes

Servings: 2

Ingredients

- 3 medium ripe avocados, halved, seeded, peeled, and cut into chunks
- 2 cloves fresh garlic, minced
- 2 cups low-sodium, fat-free chicken broth, divided
- ½ cucumber, peeled and chopped
- ½ cup chopped white onion
- ¼ cup finely diced carrot
- Thin avocado slices for garnish
- Paprika to sprinkle
- Salt and freshly ground pepper to taste
- Hot red pepper sauce to taste

Directions

1. Place 6 bowls into the freezer and allow them to chill for half an hour.
2. In the meantime, take out your blender and add garlic, cucumber, avocados, onion, carrot, and 1 cup broth. Blend all the ingredients together until they turn smooth.
3. Add the remaining broth. Add the salt and pepper and hot sauce to taste, if preferred. Blend all the ingredients again until they are smooth.
4. Take out the chilled bowls and pour the blended ingredients into them. This time, place the bowls in the refrigerator for another 1 hour.
5. When you are ready to serve, top the soup with paprika and slices of avocado. Serve chilled.

Coconut and Grilled Vegetable Soup

Preparation Time: 10 minutes

Cooking Time: 45 minutes

Servings: 4

Ingredients

- 2 small red onions cut into wedges
- 2 garlic cloves
- 10 ounces butternut squash, peeled and chopped
- 10 ounces pumpkins, peeled and chopped
- 4 tablespoons melted vegan butter
- Salt and black pepper to taste
- 1 cup of water
- 1 cup unsweetened coconut milk
- 1 lime juiced
- ¾ cup vegan mayonnaise
- Toasted pumpkin seeds for garnishing

Directions

1. Preheat the oven to 400 F.

2. On a baking sheet, spread the onions, garlic, butternut squash, and pumpkins and drizzle half of the butter on top.

3. Season with salt, black pepper, and rub the seasoning well onto the vegetables. Roast in the oven for 45 minutes or until the vegetables are golden brown and softened.

4. Transfer the vegetables to a pot; add the remaining ingredients except for the pumpkin seeds, and using an immersion blender, puree the ingredients until smooth.

5. Dish the soup, garnish with the pumpkin seeds and serve warm.

Chilled Avocado and Cucumber Soup with Basil

Preparation Time: 15 minutes + chilling time

Cooking Time: 0 minutes

Servings: 4

Ingredients

- 2 ripe avocados, pitted and peeled
- 2 large cucumbers, peeled and seeded
- 1 (13.5-ounce) can full-fat coconut milk
- 1 tablespoon lime juice
- 2 teaspoons rice vinegar
- 1 teaspoon sambal
- Kosher salt, as needed
- 1 tablespoon olive oil
- ½ cup fresh Thai or sweet basil leaves
- 1 tablespoon chopped fresh chives

Directions

1. Combine the avocado flesh, cucumber flesh, coconut milk, lime juice, rice vinegar, sambal, and salt to taste in a blender and purée until smooth.

2. If needed, pour water a tablespoon at a time to thin the mixture to the consistency of pancake batter.

3. Refrigerate the soup for at least 30 minutes or up to 3 hours.

4. Garnish each serving with a drizzle of olive oil and a sprinkle of basil and chives. Serve cold.

Apple & Kale Salad

Preparation Time: 15 minutes

Cooking Time: 15 minutes

Servings: 4

Ingredients

- 3 large apples, cored and sliced
- 6 cups fresh baby kale
- ¼ cup walnuts, chopped
- 2 tablespoons olive oil
- 1 tablespoon agave nectar
- Sea salt, as needed

Directions

1. In a salad bowl, place all ingredients and toss to coat well.
2. Serve immediately.

Orange & Kale Salad

Preparation Time: 10 minutes

Cooking Time: 10 minutes

Servings: 2

Ingredients

For the Salad:

- 3 cups fresh kale, tough ribs removed and torn
- 2 oranges, peeled and segmented
- 2 tablespoons fresh cranberries

For the Dressing:

- 2 tablespoons olive oil
- 2 tablespoons fresh orange juice
- ½ teaspoon agave nectar
- Sea salt, as needed

Directions

For the salad:

1. Place all ingredients in a salad bowl and mix.

For the dressing:

2. Place all ingredients in n another bowl and beat until well combined.
3. Pour the dressing over the salad and toss to coat well. Serve immediately.

Roasted Tomato Soup

Preparation Time: 20 mins

Cooking Time: 50 mins

Servings: 8

Ingredients

- 1 yellow onion, quartered
- 3 lbs Roma tomatoes, quartered
- ½ cup of red bell pepper, coarsely chopped
- 1 ½ tsp salt
- 3 tbsp olive oil
- 1 ½ tsp ground black pepper
- 5 cups of chicken broth, low-sodium
- 3 cloves garlic, halved
- 2 tbsp chopped fresh parsley
- 2 tbsp fresh basil, chopped

Directions

1. Preheat oven to 400 degrees F. Line 2 baking pans (10x15-inch) using parchment paper.
2. Arrange onion, bell pepper, and tomatoes in a layer on prepared baking pans. Pour the oil and sprinkle with pepper and salt.
3. Roast in a preheated oven for thirty minutes. Add the garlic; continue to roast till the mixture is tender, for about fifteen minutes more.
4. Bring the broth to boil in a big pot over a high flame. Reduce the flame and simmer, coated.
5. Meanwhile, put half of the mixture of tomato in the blender. Cover and pulse three times, blend till smooth and add the hot broth as required. Pour into pot with broth. Continue with the remaining tomato mixture; stir into pot till combined.
6. Simmer the soup to heat through for about five minutes. Mix parsley and basil.

Miso Corn Soup

Preparation Time: 10 mins

Cooking Time: 15 minutes

Servings: 2

Ingredients

- 2 tbsp of low-sodium soy sauce
- 3 oz. of tender stem broccoli, stir-fried
- 2 to 3 tbsp of oil
- 7 oz. of smoked firm tofu
- 3 oz. of vermicelli noodles, cooked
- Kernels from 2 cobs

Broth

- 2 diced garlic cloves
- 2 tsp of grated ginger
- 2 tsp of low-sodium soy sauce
- 1 tsp of toasted sesame oil
- 2 cups of veggie stock
- 1 shallot, diced
- 2 tbsp of rice wine vinegar
- 2 tbsp of white miso
- 1 tbsp of mirin

Directions

1. Cube the tofu & mix with low-sodium soy sauce, let it rest for a few minutes.
2. Sauté the ginger, shallots & garlic in hot oil for 5 minutes.
3. Mix the water (2 tbsp) with miso.
4. In a pot, add stock with miso, simmer for 10 minutes.
5. Add low-sodium soy sauce, rice wine vinegar, sesame oil & mirin.
6. Cook noodles as per package instructions.
7. Sauté the tofu in hot oil until crispy.
8. Sauté the broccoli in hot oil for 2 minutes, add kernels & cook for 2 to 3 minutes.
9. In serving bowls, add the noodles.
10. Pour the soup on top, serve with desired toppings.

Basil and Avocado Salad

Preparation Time: 10 minutes

Cooking Time: 0 minutes

Servings: 2

Ingredients

- ½ cup avocado, peeled, pitted, chopped
- ½ cup basil leaves
- ½ cup cherry tomatoes
- 2 cups cooked spelled noodles
- 1 teaspoon agave syrup
- 1 tablespoon key lime juice
- 2 tablespoons olive oil

Directions

1. Take a large bowl, place pasta in it, add tomato, avocado, and basil, and then stir until mixed.
2. Take a small bowl, add agave syrup and salt, pour in lime juice and olive oil, and then whisk until combined.
3. Pour lime juice mixture over pasta, toss until combined, and then serve.

Quinoa Salad

Preparation Time: 25 mins

Cooking Time: 20 mins

Servings: 6

Ingredients

- 1 cup of quinoa
- 2 cups of water
- ½ tsp salt, divided
- 1 baby cucumber, diced
- ½ cup of cherry tomatoes
- ¼ cup of chopped red onion
- 4 small, quartered radishes
- ¼ cup of halved Kalamata olives
- 2 tbsp olive oil
- 2 tbsp chopped fresh mint
- 2 tbsp fresh lemon juice
- 2 tbsp chopped fresh parsley
- ¼ cup of toasted diced almonds
- ¼ tsp ground black pepper

Directions

1. In a saucepan, boil the water. Add 1/4 tsp salt and 1/4 cup quinoa. Reduce the heat to a medium-low setting. Simmer, sealed, for twelve to fourteen minutes, or till quinoa is only tender and liquid has been absorbed. Remove the pan from the heat, cover, and set it aside to cool entirely.

2. Combine the tomatoes, cooled quinoa, cucumber, radishes, onion, olives, oil, mint, lemon juice, parsley, 1/4 tsp salt, and pepper in a big mixing bowl. Serve right away, or chill for up to two hours. Before serving, brush with almonds.

SNACKS

Kalamata Olive Tapenade

Preparation Time: 15 mins

Cooking Time: 0 mins

Servings: 8

Ingredients

- 1 cup of pitted kalamata olives
- 3 peeled cloves garlic
- 2 tbsp capers
- 2 tbsp lemon juice
- 3 tbsp chopped fresh parsley
- salt and pepper according to taste
- 2 tbsp olive oil

Directions

1. Put the garlic cloves into a food processor or a blender pulse to mince. Add the capers, olives, parsley, olive oil, and lemon juice. Blend till everything is chopped. Season according to taste with pepper and salt.

Kale Chips

Preparation Time: 5 minutes

Cooking Time: 15 minutes

Servings: 4

Ingredients

- 7 oz kale
- 1 tbsp coconut oil
- 1 tsp chili powder
- 1 tsp cumin

Directions

1. Warm the oven to 400 F and line a baking tray with parchment paper. Rinse the kale and allow it to dry. Tear into small pieces and discard the stems.

2. Place the kale in a mixing bowl and toss the coconut oil and spices to coat.

3. Spread the kale evenly over the baking tray and bake in the oven for 15 minutes until crispy and brown. Serve immediately.

Sesame Seed Balls

Preparation Time: 20 mins

Cooking Time: 5 mins

Servings: 12

Ingredients

- ¼ cup of oats
- 1 cup of whole wheat flour
- 3 tbsp ground flax seed
- ¼ tsp salt
- ½ tsp ground cinnamon
- ½ cup of sesame seeds
- ½ cup of honey
- ⅔ cup of crunchy peanut butter

Directions

1. In a mixing bowl, blend oats, flour, cinnamon, salt, and ground flaxseed; add peanut butter and honey and stir until well mixed. Make teaspoon-sized balls out of the mixture.

2. Pour about half of the sesame seeds into a big frying pan and toast over low heat for three to five minutes, mixing or shaking the pan every minute. Toss toasted sesame seeds into a bowl, then toast the leftover sesame seeds.

3. In a large, shallow bowl, spread the toasted seeds out. Roll them in toasted sesame seeds uniformly cover the peanut butter pieces.

Dark Chocolate and Almond Bark

Preparation Time: 20 minutes

Cooking Time: 10 minutes

Servings: 8 barks

Ingredients

- 7 oz dark chocolate (at least 75% cocoa)
- 3 1/2 oz almonds
- 2 oz pumpkin seeds
- 2 oz sunflower seeds

Directions

1. Line a baking tray with parchment paper.
2. Chop the chocolate into small pieces and place it into a heat-proof bowl. Place the bowl on top of a small saucepan filled with water.
3. Heat the saucepan to a simmer and allow the chocolate to melt, stirring occasionally.
4. When half of the chocolate has fully melted, remove the bowl from the heat and set it aside.
5. When the chocolate has cooled down slightly but is still warm, stir in the almonds, pumpkin seeds, and sunflower seeds.
6. Spread the chocolate across the lined tray and smooth the top to be even. Place in the fridge for 10-15 minutes to harden.
7. Once hardened, cut the bark into 8 servings, and enjoy.

Coconut Squares

Preparation Time: 10 minutes

Cooking Time: 30 minutes

Servings: 8

Ingredients

- 2 cups coconut flour
- 1 cup coconut flesh, unsweetened and shredded
- 1 cup walnuts, chopped
- 1 cup coconut oil
- ¼ teaspoon stevia
- Cooking spray

Directions

1. In a bowl, combine the flour with the coconut flesh and the other ingredients except for the cooking spray and stir well.

2. Spread this in a baking dish greased with the cooking spray, press well on the bottom, introduce in the oven at 350 F and bake for 30 minutes.

3. Leave aside to cool down, cut into squares and serve.

Walnut Bites

Preparation Time: 15 minutes

Cooking Time: 0 minute

Serving: 16

Ingredients

- 1 ½ cup Old Fashioned oats
- 3 tablespoons dark cocoa
- ½ teaspoon cinnamon
- 1 cup pitted soft dates
- 3 tablespoons almond butter
- 3 tablespoons dark pure maple syrup
- 3 tablespoons chopped walnuts
- 3 tablespoons mini chocolate chips

Direction:

1. Crush the oatmeal. Transfer in a bowl. Mix the cocoa, cinnamon, and salt.
2. Crush dates, add almond butter and maple syrup to make a thick paste.
3. Mold the dough to the silicone to resemble crushed cookie dough for about 2 minutes. Continue the work on the dough, and mix in the nuts and chocolate chips.
4. Knead well. Form into 14 balls. Refrigerate the refrigerator to adjust the chocolate.

Grilled Artichokes with Tarragon Butter

Preparation Time: 10 minutes

Cooking Time: 30 minutes

Servings: 2-4

Ingredients

- 2 lemons, halved
- 2 tablespoons kosher salt
- 2 tablespoons Old Bay seasoning
- 2 large globe artichokes
- 4 tablespoons (½ stick) unsalted butter
- 2 garlic cloves, minced
- 1 teaspoon minced fresh tarragon
- Grated zest of 1 lemon
- Kosher salt, as needed
- Cracked black pepper, as needed
- 1 tablespoon olive oil

Directions

1. Fill your large stockpot halfway with water and bring to a boil over high heat. Add the lemon halves, salt, and Old Bay to the boiling water.

2. Using a serrated knife, trim the top third off each artichoke. Peel the stem using a vegetable peeler, then trim the end of the stem.

3. Slice each artichoke in half lengthwise and place each in the boiling water—cover and cook within 20 minutes, or until the stems are tender. Drain and set aside.

4. Preheat an outdoor grill or cast iron stovetop grill pan on high heat.

5. Meanwhile, melt the butter in a small saucepan to make the tarragon butter. Add the garlic, tarragon, lemon zest, salt, and black pepper to taste. Keep warm on your stove until ready to serve.

6. Once the artichokes are cool enough to handle, pull the fibrous "choke" out of the middle; it should slip right out.

7. Drizzle the cut sides of the artichoke halves with the olive oil and grill them cut-side-down for 3 minutes, or until well-marked by the grill grates.

8. Serve warm with a small bowl of tarragon butter.

Coffee Walnut Bars

Preparation Time: 15 minutes

Cooking Time: 15 minutes

Servings: 14 bars

Ingredients

- 110g butter, melted
- 125ml coffee
- 60g coconut flour
- 55g walnuts, chopped
- 8 eggs
- 1 tsp baking powder
- 2 tsp vanilla
- 5 tbsp granulated sweetener
- A pinch of salt

Directions

1. Mix the butter, vanilla, and sweetener in a bowl. Add the baking powder, coconut flour, coffee, and a pinch of salt. Stir well. Add 1 egg at a time, mixing well.

2. Add the chopped walnuts. Pour the mixture into a baking dish prepared with baking paper, then bake at 356 F for 15 minutes. Once cooled, cut into 14 bars.

Oven-Roasted Brussels Sprouts

Preparation Time: 10 minutes

Cooking Time: 15-20 minutes

Servings: 4

Ingredients

- 1 pound Brussels sprouts, trimmed and halved
- 3 tablespoons extra-virgin olive oil
- Sea salt, as needed
- Freshly ground black pepper, as needed
- 1½ tablespoons balsamic vinegar

Directions

1. Preheat the oven to 375 F.
2. Toss the Brussels sprouts with the oil, then spread them out in a single layer, cut sides down on a rimmed baking sheet. Season with salt and pepper.
3. Transfer the baking sheet to the oven, and bake for 15 minutes. Drizzle the sprouts with the balsamic vinegar, tossing to coat.
4. Return the baking sheet to your oven, and bake for another 3 to 5 minutes, or until the vinegar has caramelized but not burned. Serve immediately.

Tomato & Basil Bruschetta

Preparation Time: 10 minutes

Cooking Time: 10 minutes

Servings: 3

Ingredients

- 3 tomatoes, chopped
- 1 clove garlic, minced
- ¼ tsp garlic powder (optional)
- A handful of basil leaves, coarsely chopped
- Salt, as needed
- Pepper, as needed
- ½ tsp olive oil
- ½ tbsp balsamic vinegar
- ½ tbsp butter
- ½ baguette French bread or Italian bread, sliced into ½ inch thick slices

Directions

1. Put the tomatoes, garlic, plus basil in your bowl and toss well—season with salt plus pepper. Drizzle oil plus vinegar, toss well and set aside within an hour.

2. Dissolve the butter, then brush it over your baguette slices—place in your oven and toast. Sprinkle the tomato mixture over and serve right away.

Boiled Peanuts

Preparation Time: 5 minutes

Cooking Time: 45 minutes

Servings: 4-6

Ingredients

- 2½ pounds raw, unshelled peanuts
- 1 cup salt
- 4 cups water

Directions

1. Place unshelled peanuts, salt, and water into the Instant Pot Pressure Cooker.
2. Lock the lid in place. Press the high pressure and cook for 10 minutes.
3. When the beep sounds, Choose Natural Pressure Release. Depressurizing would take 20 minutes. Remove the lid.
4. Cool before pouring to a colander. Rinse well to remove most of the salt. Drain.
5. To serve, scoop just the right number of peanuts into bowls. Shell peanuts as you eat.

Almond Paleo Date Cookies

Preparation Time: 25 mins

Cooking Time: 15 mins

Servings: 24

Ingredients

- 1 cup dates, chopped and pitted
- 1 tbsp vanilla extract
- 2 ½ cups of almond flour, blanched
- ½ cup cherries, chopped and dried
- 2 tbsp chia seeds
- ½ cup walnuts, chopped
- ½ cup of coconut oil
- ½ tsp of sea salt
- ½ tsp baking soda
- 1 egg
- 2 tbsp of maple syrup

Directions

1. Preheat your oven to 400 °F. Line two baking pans using parchment paper.

2. Whisk together dates, almond flour, cherries, chia seeds, sea salt, walnuts, and baking soda in a big mixing bowl. Blend in the egg, coconut oil, vanilla extract, and maple syrup using a fork or spoon until dough forms.

3. Using a tiny cookie scoop, spoon dough onto baking sheets.

4. Bake for fifteen minutes in a preheated oven till it gets brown from the edges. Turn off the oven and let the cookies in there for another ten minutes with the door closed. Remove from the oven and set aside to cool.

Pita Chips

Preparation Time: 15 minutes

Cooking Time: 10 minutes

Servings: 1 cup

Ingredients

- 3 pitas
- ¼ cup extra-virgin olive oil
- ¼ cup za'atar

Directions

1. Warm the oven to 450 F. Slice the pitas into 2-inch pieces, and place in your large bowl. Drizzle pitas using extra-virgin olive oil, sprinkle with za'atar, and toss until well coated.

2. Spread out pitas on your baking sheet, and bake within 8 to 10 minutes until lightly browned.

3. Let it cool before removing it from your baking sheet. Serve and enjoy!

Cauliflower Poppers

Preparation Time: 20 minutes

Cooking Time: 30 minutes

Servings: 4

Ingredients

- 4 cups cauliflower florets
- 2 teaspoons olive oil
- ¼ teaspoon chili powder
- Pepper and salt, as needed

Directions

1. Warm the oven to 450 F. Grease a roasting pan.

2. In a bowl, add all ingredients and toss to coat well.

3. Transfer the cauliflower mixture into a prepared roasting pan and spread in an even layer. Roast for about 25-30 minutes. Serve warm.

Zucchini Protein Pancakes

Preparation Time: 10 mins

Cooking Time: 5 mins

Servings: 1

Ingredients

- 1 small shredded zucchini
- ½ cup oats, old-fashioned
- 1 egg
- 1 scoop of protein powder
- 2 tbsp coconut flour
- cooking spray
- 1 tbsp stevia powder

Directions

1. In a blender, put the oats and mix them until gritty (three to four pulses). After that, move the oats to a bowl.

2. Stir egg, zucchini, coconut flour, stevia, and protein powder into oats; stir them well to make a batter.

3. Heat a pan and grease them using cooking spray. Spill the batter into the pan. Cook till the edges look dry for about three minutes. Turn and cook for another two minutes.

Protein Pumpkin Muffins

Preparation Time: 5 mins

Cooking Time: 17 mins

Servings: 24

Ingredients

- 1 ½ cups flour, all-purpose
- 2 cups protein supplement, powdered
- 1 ½ tsp salt
- 2 tsp ground cinnamon
- 2 tsp ground nutmeg
- 1 cup white sugar
- 1 ½ cups applesauce
- 1 cup vegetable oil
- 2 eggs
- 1 (15 oz) can of pumpkin puree, canned
- 2 egg whites
- 1 cup walnuts, chopped
- ½ cup water

Directions

1. Up to 350 degrees Fahrenheit, preheat your oven. Grease the muffin cups using muffin liners.

2. Mix together flour, protein powder, salt, cinnamon, sugar, and nutmeg in a bowl. Add applesauce, oil, eggs, pumpkin, water, and egg whites; mix them well.

3. Fold in walnuts, then spoon batter into the muffin cups.

4. Bake in the oven for sixteen minutes or till a toothpick placed into the middle of the muffin comes out clear.

SMOOTHIES

Blazing Broccoli Smoothie

Preparation Time: 5 minutes

Cooking Time: 0 minutes

Servings: 3-4

Ingredients

- 1 cup spinach
- 1 cup broccoli
- 1 carrot, peeled
- 1 green pepper, cored
- 1/2 lime, peeled
- 2 cups purified water

Directions

1. Combine spinach, broccoli, carrot, pepper, lime, and 1 cup of purified water in a blender and blend until thoroughly combined.

2. Add remaining water while blending until desired texture is achieved.

Recovery Smoothie

Preparation Time: 5 minutes

Cooking Time: 0 minutes

Servings: 1

Ingredients

- 1/4 banana (frozen)
- ½ cup orange juice
- ½ scoop whey protein
- 1/4 cup pineapple

Directions

1. Blend all the fixings in a blender.
2. Pour your mixture into your glass and enjoy.

Detox Support Smoothie

Preparation Time: 5 minutes

Cooking Time: 0 minutes

Servings: 2

Ingredients

- 1-2 ice cubes
- 1 cup water
- ½ avocado, chopped
- 2 carrots, chopped
- 1/2 raw beet, peeled and chopped
- 1/2 lemon, juiced

Directions

1. Combine all fixings in a high-speed blender and blend until smooth.
2. Transfer to your glasses, serve and enjoy!

Almond Kale Smoothie

Preparation Time: 5 minutes

Cooking Time: 0 minutes

Servings: 2

Ingredients

- 1 cup crushed ice, divided
- 1 cup unsweetened almond milk
- 1 cup kale
- 1 tablespoon coconut oil
- 2 tablespoons almond flour
- ½ teaspoon almond extract

Directions

1. Blend ½ cup of ice, almond milk, kale, and coconut oil in a blender.
2. Add the almond flour, almond extract, and the remaining ½ cup of ice. Blend within 1 minute, or until smooth, and serve.

Tropical Fast Smoothie

Preparation Time: 5 minutes

Cooking Time: 0 minutes

Servings: 1

Ingredients

- ½ cup kale
- ½ cup spinach
- 2 cup coconut milk
- ½ cup frozen mango
- ½ cup frozen pineapple

Directions

1. Blend the fruits and veggies in a blender.
2. Pour your mixture into your glass and enjoy.

Chamomile, Peach and Ginger Smoothie

Preparation Time: 5 minutes

Cooking Time: 0 minutes

Servings: 2

Ingredients

- 4-5 ice cubes
- 1 cup chamomile tea
- 1 lime, juiced
- 2 large peaches, chopped
- 1 tsp grated ginger

Directions

1. Combine all fixings in a high-speed blender and blend until smooth.
2. Serve and enjoy!

Mango and Cucumber Smoothie

Preparation Time: 5 minutes

Cooking Time: 0 minutes

Servings: 2

Ingredients

- 1/2 cup crushed ice or 3-4 ice cubes
- 1 cup coconut milk
- 1 mango, peeled and diced
- 1 small cucumber, peeled and chopped
- 1-2 dates, pitted
- 1 tbsp chia seeds

Directions

1. Combine all fixings in a high-speed blender and blend until smooth.
2. Serve and enjoy!

Kale and Kiwi Smoothie

Preparation Time: 5 minutes

Cooking Time: 0 minutes

Servings: 2

Ingredients

- 2-3 ice cubes
- 1 cup orange juice
- 1 small pear, peeled and chopped
- 2 kiwis, peeled and chopped
- 2-3 kale leaves
- 2-3 dates, pitted

Directions

1. Combine all fixings in a high-speed blender and blend until smooth.
2. Serve and enjoy!

Apricot, Strawberry and Banana Smoothie

Preparation Time: 5 minutes

Cooking Time: 0 minutes

Servings: 2

Ingredients

- 1 frozen banana
- 11/2 cup almond milk
- 5 dried apricots
- 1 cup fresh strawberries

Directions

1. Combine all fixings in a high-speed blender and blend until smooth.
2. Serve and enjoy!

Superfood Blueberry Smoothie

Preparation Time: 5 minutes

Cooking Time: 0 minutes

Servings: 2

Ingredients

- 2-3 cubes frozen spinach
- 1 cup green tea
- 1 banana
- 2 cups blueberries
- 1 tbsp ground flaxseed

Directions

1. Combine all fixings in a high-speed blender and blend until smooth.
2. Serve and enjoy!

Pomegranate and Fennel Smoothie

Preparation Time: 5 minutes

Cooking Time: 0 minutes

Servings: 2

Ingredients

- 1 frozen banana
- 1 cup pomegranate juice
- 1 small fennel, chopped
- 1 pear, chopped
- 1 lime, juiced

Directions

1. Combine all fixings in a high-speed blender and blend until smooth.
2. Serve and enjoy!

Ingram Content Group UK Ltd.
Milton Keynes UK
UKHW050335110723
424905UK00017B/270